LAMICTAL GUIDEBOOK

i

Dr. Pud Nielsen

Disclaimer

Lamictal (lamotrigine) is a prescription medication primarily used to treat epilepsy and bipolar disorder. Please review the following important information:

Table of Contents

INTRODUCTION TO LAMICTAL

What is Lamictal?

Lamictal (generic name: lamotrigine) is a prescription medication primarily used to treat epilepsy and bipolar disorder. It is classified as an anticonvulsant or antiepileptic drug (AED). Lamictal helps to stabilize electrical activity in the brain, thereby reducing the frequency and severity of seizures in individuals with epilepsy and helping to manage mood swings in those with bipolar disorder.

History and Development

Lamictal was developed in the late 20th century and received approval from the U.S. Food and Drug Administration (FDA) in 1994 for the treatment of epilepsy. Since its introduction, it has gained significant recognition in the medical community for its effectiveness in managing both epilepsy and bipolar disorder. Over the years,

Lamictal has become a cornerstone in the pharmacological treatment of these conditions, often chosen for its favorable side effect profile and its ability to enhance the quality of life for many patients.

The active ingredient in Lamictal, lamotrigine, works by modulating the activity of sodium channels in the brain. By inhibiting these voltage-sensitive sodium channels, lamotrigine helps to stabilize neuronal membranes, which prevents the excessive electrical activity associated with seizures and mood disorders. This mechanism makes Lamictal effective in managing:

Epilepsy: Lamictal is used to treat various types of seizures, including partial seizures, generalized seizures, and seizures associated with Lennox-Gastaut syndrome.

Bipolar Disorder: Lamictal is commonly prescribed as a mood stabilizer to help prevent episodes of depression and mania in individuals with bipolar disorder.

Importance of Lamictal in Treatment

Lamictal is often favored for its versatility and effectiveness. Unlike some other anticonvulsants and mood stabilizers, it typically has a lower risk of significant sedation or weight gain, making it a suitable option for many patients. Additionally, Lamictal can be used in conjunction with other medications, providing flexibility in treatment plans tailored to individual needs.

In summary, Lamictal is a vital medication in the management of epilepsy and bipolar disorder. Its unique mechanism of action, combined with its favorable side effect profile, has made it an important option for patients and healthcare providers alike. In the following chapters, we will explore how Lamictal works, its uses, recommended dosages, potential side effects, and guidelines for safe use.

CHAPTER ONE

How Lamictal Works

Understanding how Lamictal (lamotrigine) functions is essential for appreciating its role in treating epilepsy and bipolar disorder. This chapter will delve into its mechanism of action, the neurological processes it influences, and how it compares to other medications in its class.

Lamictal primarily works by modulating the activity of sodium channels in the brain. Here's a closer look at its action:

Sodium Channel Inhibition:

Lamotrigine binds to voltage-sensitive sodium channels, stabilizing their inactivated state. This action reduces the release of excitatory neurotransmitters, thereby decreasing neuronal excitability.

By inhibiting excessive electrical activity in the brain, Lamictal helps prevent the abnormal firing of neurons that leads to seizures.

Neurotransmitter Modulation:

In addition to its effects on sodium channels, lamotrigine also influences the release of several neurotransmitters, including glutamate and aspartate. These neurotransmitters are often involved in seizure activity and mood regulation.

By balancing neurotransmitter levels, Lamictal can help stabilize mood and reduce the frequency of both manic and depressive episodes in bipolar disorder.

Indications for Use

Lamictal is prescribed for several conditions, primarily:

Epilepsy:

It is effective in treating various types of seizures, including partial seizures (with or without secondary generalization) and generalized seizures (such as tonic-clonic seizures). It is also approved for use in patients with Lennox-Gastaut syndrome, a severe form of epilepsy.

Bipolar Disorder:

Lamictal is utilized as a mood stabilizer, particularly effective in preventing episodes of depression and mania. It is often used in combination with other medications to achieve optimal mood stabilization.

Comparison with Other Antiepileptic Drugs

Unique Mechanism: Unlike many other antiepileptic drugs that primarily enhance inhibitory neurotransmission (like GABA), Lamictal's mechanism centers on inhibiting excitatory neurotransmission and stabilizing neuronal membranes.

Side Effect Profile: Lamictal is generally well-tolerated, with a lower incidence of sedation, weight gain, and cognitive impairment compared to some other antiepileptic medications. This makes it a favorable option for many patients.

Dosing and Titration

Due to the risk of serious skin reactions, such as Stevens-Johnson syndrome, Lamictal requires careful titration. The dosage is gradually increased to minimize potential side effects and ensure optimal therapeutic levels.

Lamictal works primarily by inhibiting sodium channels and modulating neurotransmitter release, effectively stabilizing electrical activity in the brain. This mechanism underpins its effectiveness in treating epilepsy and mood disorders.

Understanding how Lamictal functions helps patients and healthcare providers make informed decisions about its use. In the next chapter, we will explore the various uses of Lamictal in more detail, including indications and off-label applications.

CHAPTER TWO

Uses of Lamictal

Lamictal (lamotrigine) is a versatile medication primarily used to manage epilepsy and bipolar disorder. Its unique mechanism of action and favorable side effect profile make it an important option in these conditions. This chapter explores the specific uses of Lamictal, its indications, and some off-label applications.

1. Treatment of Epilepsy

Lamictal is primarily indicated for the treatment of epilepsy, and it is effective in managing various seizure types:

Partial Seizures: Lamictal is effective in controlling partial seizures, which can be simple (without loss of consciousness) or complex (with impaired consciousness). It helps reduce the frequency and severity of these seizures.

Generalized Seizures: It is also used to manage generalized tonic-clonic seizures, which involve loss of consciousness and muscle stiffening or jerking.

Lennox-Gastaut Syndrome: Lamictal is approved for use in patients with Lennox-Gastaut syndrome, a severe form of epilepsy characterized by multiple seizure types and cognitive impairment. It can help reduce the frequency of seizures associated with this condition.

Adjunctive Therapy: Lamictal can be used as an adjunctive treatment alongside other antiepileptic medications. This combination approach may be necessary for patients who do not achieve adequate seizure control with monotherapy.

2. Management of Bipolar Disorder

Lamictal is commonly prescribed as a mood stabilizer for individuals with bipolar disorder:

Prevention of Mood Episodes: Lamictal is particularly effective in preventing depressive episodes in bipolar disorder, making it valuable for long-term management. It helps stabilize mood and can mitigate the risk of both manic and depressive episodes.

Mood Stabilization: While it is not typically used to treat acute manic episodes, it can provide stabilization in patients with mixed features or those transitioning between depressive and manic phases.

3. Off-Label Uses

In addition to its approved indications, Lamictal has several off-label uses, which include:

Depression: Some clinicians use Lamictal as an adjunctive treatment for major depressive disorder, particularly in cases where traditional antidepressants are insufficient.

Anxiety Disorders: Lamictal may be utilized in managing anxiety disorders, especially when co-occurring with mood disorders.

Neuropathic Pain: Lamictal is sometimes prescribed for certain types of neuropathic pain, leveraging its effects on neuronal excitability.

Lamictal is a versatile medication primarily indicated for the treatment of epilepsy and bipolar disorder. Its ability to manage various seizure types and stabilize mood makes it a critical tool in psychiatric and neurological care. Additionally, its off-label uses highlight its potential benefits in other conditions, although these should always be approached with caution and under medical guidance. In the next chapter, we will explore the available forms of Lamictal and recommended dosages for effective treatment.

CHAPTER THREE

Dosage and Administration of Lamictal

Correct dosing and administration are crucial for maximizing the effectiveness of Lamictal (lamotrigine) while minimizing the risk of side effects. This chapter provides an overview of the available forms of Lamictal, recommended dosages, and guidelines for administration.

Available Forms

Lamictal is available in several formulations:

Tablets: Standard immediate-release tablets come in various strengths (e.g., 25 mg, 50 mg, 100 mg, 200 mg).

Chewable Tablets: These are designed for easier administration, especially for those who may have difficulty swallowing pills (available in 2 mg and 5 mg).

Orally Disintegrating Tablets: These dissolve on the tongue, providing an alternative for those who prefer not to swallow tablets (available in 25 mg and 50 mg).

Extended-Release Tablets: These are designed for once-daily dosing and are available in strengths of 100 mg, 200 mg, and 300 mg.

The dosage of Lamictal varies based on the condition being treated, the patient's age, and whether it is used alone or in combination with other medications. Below are general guidelines:

Titration: Increase by 25 mg to 50 mg every 1 to 2 weeks, based on clinical response.

Maintenance Dose: The effective dose is usually between 100 mg and 200 mg per day, depending on individual response.

3. Dosing Adjustments

Patients Taking Valproate: If a patient is also taking valproate (another anticonvulsant), the dose of Lamictal may need to be reduced, as valproate increases lamotrigine levels.

Patients Taking Other Medications: When used with other medications that induce hepatic enzymes (such as carbamazepine), the dose of Lamictal may need to be increased.

With or Without Food: Lamictal can be taken with or without food, although consistency is key. Taking it the same way each time can help maintain stable drug levels.

Missed Dose: If a dose is missed, it should be taken as soon as remembered unless it is almost time for the next dose. In that case, skip the missed dose and resume the regular dosing schedule. Do not double up on doses.

Discontinuation: Abruptly stopping Lamictal can increase the risk of seizures. It is important to taper the dosage under the supervision of a healthcare provider.

The appropriate dosing and administration of Lamictal are critical to its effectiveness and safety. Following the recommended guidelines for dosages based on the condition being treated and individual patient factors can help optimize treatment outcomes. In the next chapter, we will explore the benefits of Lamictal, highlighting its efficacy in managing epilepsy and bipolar disorder.

CHAPTER FOUR

Benefits of Lamictal

Lamictal (lamotrigine) offers several advantages for individuals dealing with epilepsy and bipolar disorder. Understanding these benefits can help patients and healthcare providers make informed decisions about treatment options. This chapter outlines the key benefits of Lamictal, including its efficacy, safety profile, and unique features.

1. Efficacy in Seizure Control

Wide Range of Seizure Types: Lamictal is effective in treating various types of seizures, including partial seizures, generalized tonic-clonic seizures, and seizures associated with Lennox-Gastaut syndrome. This broad spectrum makes it suitable for many patients with epilepsy.

Reduced Frequency of Seizures: Clinical studies have demonstrated that Lamictal significantly reduces the frequency of seizures in patients, improving their overall quality of life and allowing them to engage in daily activities with greater confidence.

Adjunctive Therapy: For patients not achieving adequate seizure control with monotherapy, Lamictal can be used in combination with other antiepileptic drugs, providing an effective adjunct to existing treatment regimens.

2. Mood Stabilization in Bipolar Disorder

Prevention of Mood Episodes: Lamictal is particularly effective in preventing depressive episodes in individuals with bipolar disorder. It helps stabilize mood and reduces the risk of cycling between manic and depressive phases.

Minimal Sedation: Unlike some mood stabilizers and antidepressants, Lamictal typically does not cause sedation or cognitive impairment, allowing individuals to maintain a clear mind and daily functioning.

Long-Term Management: Lamictal can be an effective option for long-term mood stabilization, helping patients manage their condition over time with fewer side effects compared to some alternative treatments.

3. Favorable Side Effect Profile

Low Risk of Weight Gain: Many patients appreciate that Lamictal is associated with a low risk of weight gain, which can be a concern with other medications used for mood stabilization and seizure management.

Well-Tolerated: Clinical studies indicate that Lamictal is generally well-tolerated, with a side effect profile that is manageable for most patients. Common side effects, such as headache or dizziness, are often mild and transient.

Skin Reactions: While serious skin reactions can occur, they are rare, particularly with careful titration of the dose. Patients who follow dosing guidelines are less likely to experience these adverse effects.

4. Flexibility in Treatment

Multiple Formulations: Lamictal is available in various forms, including standard tablets, chewable tablets, and orally disintegrating tablets, making it easier for patients to adhere to their treatment regimen, especially those who may have difficulty swallowing pills.

Tailored Dosing: The ability to adjust dosages and combine Lamictal with other medications allows healthcare providers to tailor treatment plans to meet the unique needs of each patient.

5. Positive Impact on Quality of Life

Enhanced Daily Functioning: By effectively managing seizures and stabilizing mood, Lamictal can significantly improve a patient's ability to participate in daily activities, work, and maintain relationships.

Improved Overall Well-Being: Patients often report a greater sense of well-being and reduced anxiety regarding their condition, thanks to the effectiveness of Lamictal in managing their symptoms.

Lamictal offers numerous benefits for individuals with epilepsy and bipolar disorder, including effective seizure control, mood stabilization, a favorable side effect profile, and flexibility in treatment options. These advantages contribute to improved quality of life and greater confidence in managing these conditions. In the next chapter, we will discuss the potential side effects associated with Lamictal, ensuring that patients are fully informed about their treatment options.

Potential Side Effects of Lamictal
While Lamictal (lamotrigine) is generally well-tolerated and effective for treating epilepsy and bipolar disorder, like any medication, it can cause

side effects. Understanding these potential side effects is essential for patients and healthcare providers to manage them appropriately. This chapter outlines the common, serious, and rare side effects associated with Lamictal.

1. Common Side Effects

Many patients taking Lamictal experience mild side effects, which often improve with continued use or dosage adjustments. Common side effects include:

Headache: A frequent complaint among users, headaches may occur but are usually manageable with over-the-counter pain relief.

Dizziness: Some patients may feel lightheaded or dizzy, particularly when starting the medication or increasing the dosage.

Nausea: Gastrointestinal discomfort, including nausea, can occur, though it is generally mild.

Fatigue: Some individuals report feeling unusually tired or fatigued while on Lamictal.

Rash: Skin rashes are relatively common but can vary in severity. Most rashes are mild and resolve with discontinuation of the medication.

2. Serious Side Effects

Although rare, Lamictal can lead to more severe side effects, which require immediate medical attention:

Stevens-Johnson Syndrome (SJS): This is a severe skin reaction characterized by flu-like symptoms followed by a painful rash that can blister and peel. It is potentially life-threatening and requires immediate discontinuation of the drug.

Toxic Epidermal Necrolysis (TEN): A more severe form of skin reaction than SJS, TEN involves widespread skin peeling and can be fatal.

Aseptic Meningitis: In rare cases, patients may experience inflammation of the protective membranes covering the brain and spinal cord, presenting with symptoms like headache, fever, and stiff neck.

Blood Dyscrasias: Lamictal may cause changes in blood cell counts, leading to conditions like thrombocytopenia (low platelet count) or leukopenia (low white blood cell count). Symptoms can include unexplained bruising, bleeding, or increased infections.

3. Rare Side Effects

Some side effects of Lamictal occur infrequently but should still be monitored:

Coordination Problems: Some patients may experience difficulties with balance or coordination.

Mood Changes: While Lamictal stabilizes mood in bipolar disorder, some individuals may experience mood swings or worsening depression, particularly when initiating or adjusting the dose.

4. Managing Side Effects

Monitoring: Regular follow-ups with healthcare providers are crucial for monitoring side effects, especially during the initial treatment phase or when adjusting doses.

Titration: Gradually increasing the dose can help minimize the risk of side effects, particularly severe skin reactions.

Immediate Reporting: Patients should be educated about the signs of serious side effects, especially skin reactions, and should report any concerning symptoms immediately.

While Lamictal is an effective treatment option for epilepsy and bipolar disorder, it is essential to be aware of potential side effects, both common and serious. By understanding these risks and maintaining open communication with healthcare providers, patients can manage their treatment effectively and safely. In the next chapter, we will discuss guidelines for the safe use of Lamictal, including important considerations for patients and healthcare providers.

Lifestyle and Management Strategies for Lamictal Users

Integrating lifestyle changes and management strategies can significantly enhance the effectiveness of Lamictal (lamotrigine) in treating epilepsy and bipolar disorder. This chapter explores various approaches to support overall health, improve medication adherence, and manage the conditions effectively.

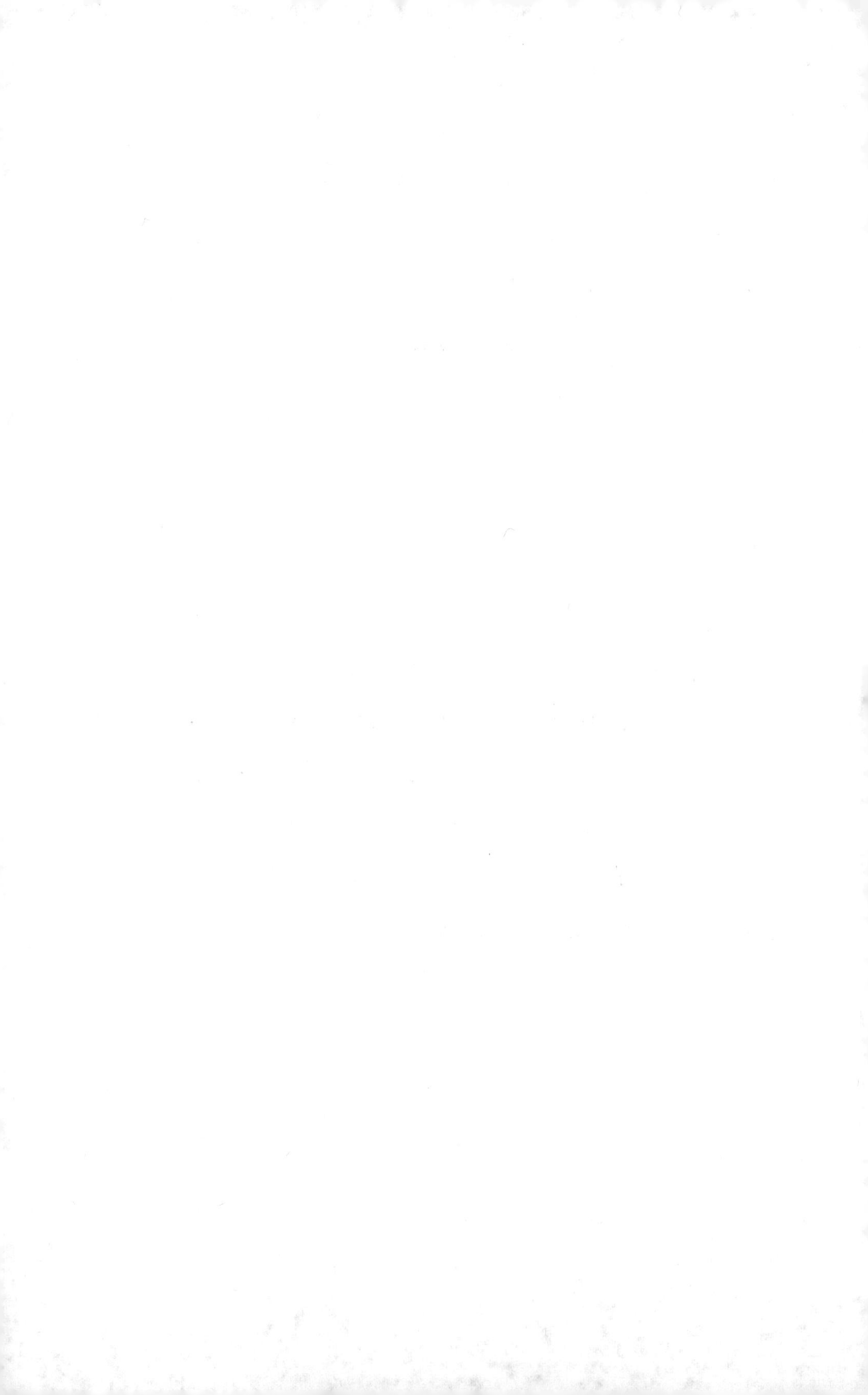

9 7 9 8 3 4 1 1 3 2 3 4 4